DEAR CHRONIC
ILLNESS

COMPILED BY
PIPPA STACEY

DEAR CHRONIC ILLNESS

First published in 2018
by Wallace Publishing, United Kingdom
www.wallacepublishing.co.uk

Typesetting courtesy of KGHH Publishing, United Kingdom
www.kensingtongorepublishing.com

CONTENTS

ABOUT SPOONIE SURVIVAL KITS

Spoonie Survival Kits first began as a small fundraising project, whereby twenty 'Little Bags of Happiness' were created, designed with those suffering from chronic illnesses in mind. The kits initially contained things to do, make, eat and wear, in the hope of providing comfort to recipients and making their tough days a little more bearable.

The kits were sold online, with the money raised from sales being donated to charity. The chronic illness community's overwhelmingly positive response to this small initiative allowed the project to grow considerably, becoming a non-profit fundraising project. The kits continued to be made and distributed, hitting fundraising targets for a variety of causes. These have so far included registered charities supporting those with chronic illnesses, including Myalgic Encephalomyelitis, Fibromyalgia, POTS and Ehlers-Danlos Syndrome, as well as non-profit initiatives such as Project Parent UK. We strive to fundraise for as many worthy causes as possible, and at the time of writing, have raised nearly £4000 in total.

Due to an ever-increasing demand for our goodies, Spoonie Survival Kits is currently under reform again, this time being transformed and upgraded into a social enterprise. This upscaling has allowed us to create accessible volunteering opportunities for those with long-term illnesses, and even set our sights on possible employment opportunities for this population in the future. Our kits contain items made by talented crafters with disabilities and chronic illnesses, and we've also created opportunities in graphic design, web design and administration for the incredibly kind-hearted people who have come forward and asked what they could do to help our cause. We currently have a wonderful little family working diligently on making Spoonie Survival Kits the very best it can be, and we can't wait to see what the future holds for us!

FIBROMYALGIA- ADRIEL MADONADO

Dear Fibromyalgia,

You and I have been together so long, I don't even know for sure when you first entered my life.

Was it you that caused that excruciating pain that everyone said was growing pains when I was seven? Was it you that drained my energy so quickly and easily? Was it you, fibromyalgia, that prevented me from having a normal childhood?

I may never know the answer to that. But I do know it was you that reared your ugly head when I was merely a teen. While other young ones my age were having the time of their life, I was constantly saving my energy for only the most important things.

It was you, fibromyalgia, which left me in so much pain, day in and day out. It was you that caused debilitating fatigue, no matter how much I slept. Because of you I missed out on so much. Because of you, I genuinely thought I was dying.

I hoped with all of my might that if I ignored you, you would eventually go away. I would have times when I thought you were gone. But you always came back.

I tried so hard to hide the damage you were causing. I didn't want anyone knowing the pain you inflicted. I was convinced they would think I was making you up. I was worried that they may treat me differently. So I hid you, like a dirty secret.

The time came that I could no longer hide you. You were taking over my life and I just couldn't ignore you anymore.

I had just gotten married to a wonderful man and I was the happiest I had ever been. But you didn't care. You struck me again, hard and heavy.

The doctor felt sure it was you. After lots of testing, I was told he was right. I had just turned twenty-two and was in the prime of my life but here I was, being told I would be sick for the rest of my life.

"It won't kill you," the doctor assured me, "but the pain may make you wish it would." I was shocked a doctor would say such a thing, but he wasn't wrong.

Because of you, I have been on and off of multiple medications, vitamins, supplements, and diets. I have spent a countless amount of money paying for doctors and treatments. So much money that my family could have used for other things, money that might as well have been flushed down the toilet.

You have inserted yourself so fully into my life that sometimes I don't know where you end and I begin. You influence my thinking, my decision-making, and worst of all, my relationships.

What could my husband and I have done together if you weren't around? Would we have traveled the world? Would we have spent our time helping others? Would we have spent our time going to concerts and going out dancing? I guess we will never know.

What kind of mom could I have been had you not forced yourself upon me? Would I have taken my boys to the park every day? Would I have spent hours playing with them? Would I have made all their food from scratch, ensuring they grew up strong and healthy? I will never know.

What could I have become? Who could I have helped? What things could I have made or spent my time doing if you were not a part of my life?

With you in my life, I have to spend my days sitting, moving as little as possible so that I have the strength to take care of the most important things.

You are always on my mind. Even when you give me a brief reprieve, you still haunt me because I know you will come back. I know that in this life, I will never be completely rid of you.

Sometimes it feels like you hate me, like you want to make me miserable. It feels like a deliberate, personal attack against me and my happiness.

I have to admit though, it hasn't been all bad. Because of you I discovered a whole new community and support group. I found that I was not alone.

Because of you, I have learned to be more sympathetic and sensitive to the suffering of others.

You have helped me to discover what is truly important in life. I now have a better understanding that who you are as a person is what really matters.

I am able to better appreciate the little things in life. I have learned to never take small acts of kindness and friendship for granted. I have learned to be gracious, to be content, and to be patient.

I have learned a lot about myself. I have seen how I respond to the darkest of days. I have seen myself hit rock bottom, but not give up. I have seen myself come dangerously close to giving up, but I haven't, and I know that I won't.

Because you are a part of my life, I know that I am stronger than I ever thought possible. I am a survivor. I am a warrior.

I have learned to accept you. I will never stop fighting for the best life possible for me and my family, but I also know that I cannot fight you. I know I have to accept that you are a part of my life and learn how to make the best of what I have.

Whether I like it or not, you will always be a part of my life. You have shaped my life and for good or bad, you have shaped the person that I am.

You have definitely changed my life, but I have learned not all change is a bad thing.

Love,
Adriel

ENDOMETRIOSIS – AIMEE FINLAY

Dear Endometriosis,

I know I complain about your presence in my life, but almost three years after my diagnosis, I have finally found our silver lining! You took your sweet time, but I finally found it!

As you know, for us ladies with Endometriosis, living life as normally as possible is a struggle. With chronic pain so severe and heavy irregular periods, it is easy for life to get us down.

After I've had a sucky time and I am over the initial trauma of an appointment, a diagnosis, and surgery, I try to find something about it to laugh at. I know I shouldn't because illness is serious, but I regularly use this as a coping mechanism and it makes light of my illness.

I guess humour can be as uplifting as opioids, if you use it properly!

And so, this is the first of many **LOL** moments. Be assured that I will spare no details, no matter how embarrassing, and I hope to hell you don't judge me. Enjoy!

Last week, on a grey morning, I woke up with a sad feeling. I was grumpy and just couldn't brush it off. There's no point in dressing this up as something else. I was mardy and tired and feeling sorry for myself. So I tried my cure-all, feel-better Go-To's:

- I had a cup of tea and dunker biscuits in bed, which has always sorted me out in the past – but no.

- I watched the original Ghostbusters film (Remember? Bill Murray is a sure way to make me smile). Nope.

- I had a scalding hot bath with a Lush bath bomb. I soaked until I was pruney & short of breath from the steam… Nothing.

- With determination we'd not seen in weeks, I got out of the bath and dressed quickly. Trying to put socks on and hold my phone to my ear is not easy and, being clumsy like I am, I stumbled more than once as I waited for my mum to answer her phone.

"Mum, it's me – Yeah, no, I'm fine – I need you to come get me – Soon, like ten minutes? – We're going to town, to King's – I need to buy a bag."

As you can see, this needed action. This mood had to do one. And in order for that to happen, I needed a handbag. My mum (being the treasure that she is) dropped everything.

Mum and I went to a local boutique-with-café in my town and I immediately headed for the bag section. Usually, it is chocker with homeware and ornaments- things that I'd break just looking at them. But at this time, the owners were making way for their Christmas stock. That in itself was exciting! It's like a frigging grotto in there every Christmas, and it would soon be time to put my tree up! This lightened my mood considerably and I hadn't even set my sights on a single bag yet.

Then I found her. She was an Anna Smith tote. I carried her around the shop like a small baby while I browsed. I held her in my lap as I waited for coffee. I paid £42 for her and that was money-well-spent as far as I was concerned!

There is nothing more satisfying for a bag-lover, than transferring your things out of your old bag and into a new one. I filled all the pockets with my stuff, forgetting that in a month, everything would be dumped in and I'd have to wade through a pile of old receipts and wrappers and leaflets.

I needed this bag. Not only to make me feel better, but since I now have to take a ton of stuff with me everywhere I go, I needed a bigger, hardier bag. Obviously, I had all the usual suspects: purse, keys, glasses, pen, notebook, diary, gum, and perfume/deodorant. But now that I have a reproductive system with a mind of its own, I also have to carry: about three-thousand pads, a heat pad, spare knickers, and a small pouch of pain meds (which I'm sure would get me arrested if I was searched by police!)

I can fit all my baggage into this tote bag. Just call me Mary Poppins.

It can be hard being a girl. But it's a nightmare being a girl with Endometriosis.

We deserve handbags. *Thank you*, Anna Smith, for helping me find the brighter side.

So Endo, bye for now, until next month's flare.

Chronically yours,

Aimee & her fabulous new bag x

M.E – PIPPA STACEY

Dear M.E,

If this letter was part of an inspirational movie, I'm sure I would be saying a heartfelt thank you. Dramatic music would play whilst I'd gush about how becoming ill changed my life for the better and helped me discover more about myself as a person, whilst I waltzed off into the sunset with a handsome prince and some kind of small fortune due to a dramatic plot twist.

Unfortunately, this is not an inspirational movie. Instead of waltzing off into the sunset, I manoeuvre an unreliable wheelchair along a questionably uneven pavement. Instead of finding a handsome prince, I concentrate on finding the most qualified medical professionals to manage my condition… with bonus points if they happen to be attractive, of course. And my plot twist isn't a small fortune: it's not knowing if, when or how I will ever get better.

As a classical ballet dancer in training, I grew up learning that in order to succeed in my vocation, I had to push my body beyond its physical limits and never let up, not even for a second. When I first became poorly at the age of fifteen, my natural instinct was to adopt this same approach. By mentally squashing down my symptoms as best as I could and pushing on through, I thought my body would remember that people like me don't get ill… people like me don't have the time for that. Although this was a truly destructive approach, it was at first not only reinforced but also commended by my childhood GP. I was encouraged to increase my stamina even further, despite the fact I'd been training for up to ten hours a day for most of my life.

Although I was only mildly ill at this point, the next four years saw a slow but steady increase in symptoms. At the time, I was so focused on GCSEs, A-Levels, and throwing myself wholeheartedly into my first year of university that it wasn't at all obvious that my health was deteriorating, not even to myself. It was at the age of nineteen that my body broke down and my goodness, it didn't hold back. I was knocked down by a sudden onset of debilitating fatigue and pain attacks, orthostatic intolerance, chest pain, endless migraines, extreme sensitivity to noise and light, cognitive function difficulties, and much more. Naturally, because life is never simple, I was in Greece in a holiday resort employed as a nanny at the time. It was only after returning home and becoming confined to my bed, unable to care for myself, that I was finally referred to a specialist. They rigorously assessed me, and then diagnosed me with M.E.

Now, the typical understanding of modern medicine implies that after the diagnosis of a debilitating disease, a plan is made and treatment is begun. The problem here is that a fluctuating disease like M.E is not something that progresses along a set path. A lack of research means that as of now, there is no prognosis, targeted treatment or cure for the condition. So off I went back to my dark, quiet room at home, wondering where exactly things would go from here. For many people with M.E, this stage of uncertainty is where they have remained for years. They've been diagnosed with the condition and discharged, sometimes decades ago, and haven't been able to leave their homes, or even their beds, ever since.

Fortunately, I was one of the luckier ones. I made small improvements over time and, with plenty of support and adjustments, was able to return to university. Although my university experience from this point onwards was much more diluted, it was a real privilege to carry on living independently. I couldn't leave the house often but worked hard from my bed, received domestic care to help manage household tasks, and even maintained something of a social life. In case you're wondering, being a student with a chronic illness is a whole other world: attempting to conduct trips out in my wheelchair as I'm pushed by housemates in heels, on cobbles, after cocktails, has been a battle in its own right, as has learning how to swallow medication whilst wearing red lipstick. I graduated in 2016 with a degree in Psychology, and I hope to work with those affected by long-term illness in the future.

Although I still suffer a great deal with you, M.E, my health has continued to slowly improve. I'm more than aware that I'm one of the more fortunate ones and I couldn't appreciate the health I have more. However, throughout this whole ordeal, I couldn't help but notice what a lack of support there was for people like me. There are hundreds and hundreds of programmes and schemes for teens and young adults in hospitals, which are absolutely wonderful and play a much-needed supportive role in improving the patients' quality of life. But what about the thousands of patients suffering at home, behind closed doors, some of who are too severely unwell to even tolerate being in hospital? I had a good old think about this during all my hours in bed, and came up with the idea of Spoonie Survival Kits: 'spoonie' being the slang word for a chronic illness sufferer.

I created little bags of happiness that would endeavour to remind patients that they are not alone, that they haven't been forgotten, and that somebody is thinking of them. I decided to sell these kits online, so that everybody who wanted one could order their own, and I wanted to donate a percentage of sales money to chronic illness charities. I was genuinely shocked by the support and backing my idea received from the chronic illness community, and suddenly found myself running a social enterprise, mostly from my bed. Since then, the project has gone from strength-to-strength, by increasing awareness of debilitating long-term conditions and raising thousands of pounds for various chronic illness charities.

The support of others has been the most humbling thing of all: patients all over the world, even those so severely ill that they cannot leave their beds, have come forward to ask what they can do to help. I've found that many of these people are too unwell to work or study themselves, but they do want to use what little strength they have to volunteer. Due to the nature of fluctuating conditions, it can be immensely difficult to find appropriate opportunities with understanding employers. This has led to what I feel is Spoonie Survival Kits' biggest asset: offering accessible volunteering opportunities to fellow sufferers. We offer flexible roles that can be pursued remotely with no time constraints, stress or pressure. So far, we've provided opportunities in graphic design, administration and website maintenance, as well as recruiting plenty of experienced crafters to help us fill our kits. Not only does the enterprise benefit from having such talented, kind-hearted people involved, but it adds a special touch to our kits: our recipients are often so pleased to know that their kit contains items made especially for people with chronic illnesses, by those in similar situations. I'm so immensely grateful to everybody who's ever worked on the project, donated money or resources, or even simply spread the word about what we're doing: I truly couldn't have done it without you. At the time of writing, we're actually making some pretty drastic changes to Spoonie Survival Kits, to upscale and cope with our ever-increasing demand, but I hope we continue to raise money and awareness, and connect chronic illness sufferers all over the world. I can't wait to see where we go from here.

So I suppose this is the point where the dramatic music

would begin and I'd launch into a passionate speech about how glad I am to have become ill. I have so much respect for people who feel this way but I have to be honest: I'm not that person and I never will be. I still suffer a great deal and I am desperate to be better again. I want nothing more than for M.E to finally gain the recognition and research it warrants, and for all patients to access the care they deserve. However, I will say this: I'd like to thank you, M.E, for opening my eyes. Without becoming so poorly, I wouldn't have seen how many people are silently suffering, and how little support is in place for them. I wouldn't be running a social enterprise in my Disney pyjamas. I wouldn't have known just how powerful young people, even critically-ill young people, can be in bringing about much-needed social change. So for that, I suppose I really should say a reluctant thank you. Now, dear M.E, please feel free to bugger off and leave me alone on my mission to help Spoonie Survival Kits conquer the world of chronic illness. That would be a plot twist I really could get on board with.

Yours (but hopefully not forever),
Pippa x

EHLERS-DANLOS SYNDROME – BETHAN GRIFFITH-SALTER

Dear Ehlers-Danlos Syndrome,

It's safe to say you've made my life pretty interesting. There's been countless hospital trips and a lot of hours spent in bed with many ups-and-downs and a few tears in between. However, I would not be the person I am today without you and there have been so many laughs at your expense, as well as amazing opportunities. I have got some great stories because of you and they're always crowd-pleasers. I mean, it's because of you making me look so damn young that I was I.D'd for Bonjela and nail varnish remover. Plus, how many people can say they had to go to hospital due to an injury from eating a cereal bar or that they ended up in a sling from playing ring-a-roses? There is never a dull moment with you around.

University was probably some of the toughest years of my life. Every time I thought I had got a grip on everything, you pulled the rug out from under me again. I swear you waited until I was drowning in assignments to bless me with a massive flare. The friends I made, and the experiences and memories I gained, more than made up for it. There was that night out where I bandaged up my dislocated knee because I wanted to party instead of going to A&E. It didn't seem like such a good idea the next day, when we had to spend four hours in A&E with a hangover.

Will my mum ever let me forget the time I fell out of my

wheelchair wrapped in a curtain after a few too many drinks? Probably not. Also, let's not forget that time I tried to go round the Welsh Mountain Zoo in my wheelchair. The clue's kinda in the title that it's not exactly the best place to take a wheelchair. Then there was that time I laughed so hard that I dislocated a rib and my friends were so grossed out, I couldn't stop laughing long enough to put it back.

The fact that you won't let me write and make concentrating impossible meant that I met one of my best friends. I was so lucky that my note taker was one of the loveliest, most supportive people I've ever met. Not only did I survive uni despite you but it made graduating with a 2:1 in Biomedical Science so much sweeter. Plus I didn't have to walk in my heels and I didn't get my graduation gown caught in my wheelchair wheels, so it was an all-round success.

Travelling with you isn't the easiest but it really is fun. Attempting to use public transport in Berlin, Nice and Barcelona was definitely entertaining. I was not a fan of the huge amount of cobbles in Berlin though. I didn't think my joints would ever stop rattling. It would also seem some people aren't so used to seeing a girl with pink hair in a wheelchair, so we got some beautiful looks. Then there was that Dutch guy who tried to bless you away and wished me a speedy recovery. I'll never forget the view from the top of that hill in Monaco either, even though it took three of us to push my chair up there. Then there was that one in Barcelona, where we discovered the cable car that would've taken us from the train station to the top, after we'd already reached the top. I thought you were going to finish me off that day but the view and the laugh was worth it.

Finishing uni and being constantly asked what I was going to do with my life was a tad scary. You made it impossible to get dressed some days, let alone get a full-time job. You have, however, taught me how to adapt. You encouraged me to start a blog and I am so happy you did.

Even the name was inspired by you, because obviously, Mermaids have to use wheelchairs on land. I'm pretty damn proud of Mermaid in Disguise and you make it a better place. You inspire so much content and we can do it from the comfort of my bed. You've inspired me to be more creative and do more of what I love, like buying so much makeup. That's for the blog... obviously.

After hating you for making me give up gymnastics as a child, not being allowed to do P.E at school, and never really being active, who would've thought that I would spend every weekend competing or training? Wheelchair basketball seems to have taken over my life and I'm surprised to say I love it. Obviously you still make yourself known but the injuries and aches and pains are definitely worth it. Plus, my tape and supports collection is pretty damn impressive at the moment. I've competed for wales, recently won our division at Women's League and have made some amazing friends. I'm not really enjoying the dislocated shoulder and elbow from my spectacular fall the other week though. Thanks for keeping me in my place.

One of the best things about you though, is all the friends I have made. There are so many genuinely lovely and amazing people that I have only "met" through our weird bodies. There is always someone at the touch of a button to chat and laugh with. I've made some of my closest friends online because of you. I love that and could not be more grateful to you. You have also brought me closer to my family and we get to spend so much quality time at family doctors for appointment outings. Thanks for making me the weird and wonderful person I am today.

Much Love

Bethan

M.E – ELIZABETH GUNTRIP

Dear Myalgic Encephalomyelitis (M.E. /CFS),
You have made me stay indoors today, M.E. It's too cold out there this evening. From where I'm sitting by the window, I can see the sun's rays already leaving the sky. The traffic roars in the street below; people caught in the rat race, hurrying from place to place. I was one of them too, once. It feels like a lifetime ago.

I still remember my old way of life, before everything changed and you came into my world. Back then, I was just a confused seventeen-year-old girl; the paths I trod – of convention, of normality – were well-worn, filled with people doing the same. Life was about good luck and endless competition.

I didn't see you, at first. I didn't know about chronic illness and so you crept up on me. But you hit me – and then you stuck around. Your grip was fierce and unwavering. Myalgic Encephalomyelitis, you are tenacious.

The world with you in it, M.E., was so different. Life's paths were no longer predetermined, the ground beneath my feet unknown. Time beat with a different pulse, and it echoed in me too. My life was slower and consisted of many rests and breaks – the world could seem very quiet in a body without strength or energy.

It was during these endless hours alone that I started to recognise the little things in the world around me. I watched the sunlit rain through the window; I listened to the birds singing outside my London home; I noted the wind raking the trees – these things shone bright and true, like islands of light in the wilderness. I started to live for such moments of joy. My existence – no longer defined by mainstream achievement and success – became filled with the celebration of life's daily wonders. I learned to appreciate it all.

I explored this new way of life. I uncovered new skills and strengths, as well as dreams I had once left behind in favour of mainstream pursuits. Myalgic Encephalomyelitis, could you have guessed I would find things I could still do, and not focus on what you had taken from me? I wrote stories and read books and poetry; I learned about cars and coding and broadcasting; I even mastered the creation of pretty folded origami geese! I cradled the things I had, holding them close, these simple treasures.

You can be funny, you know, Myalgic Encephalomyelitis. Sometimes, when you get into my brain, you switch words around: coats are goats or boats, whilst radiators become 'those squiggly metal things that get hot'. Out in the wider world, you make my life even stranger. In galleries, I've faked interest in the direst of paintings because of their proximity to a chair. I've had late night conversations with the furniture because I hadn't the strength to open my eyes and see my friend had wandered off for a cup of tea. I laugh at these little slip-ups, but I'm not laughing at myself. I'm laughing at you. We are not the same.

And that was how I built myself back up from what you did to me. The ashes of my former existence proved fertile and I made myself into the best person I could be now: someone who was more open, honest, and wise. I was gentler, more patient (occasionally) and always more kind. Life can be so unpredictable and difficult and cruel, but in seeking the beauty in the world around me, in holding on to my dreams and persevering through hardship, I became so much more than my illness. My inner self, my identity, prevailed – and it ran deep and strong and pure.

Night is now falling and everything will soon be still. Tomorrow, the rest of the world will get back up and head out into the rat race yet again. Those people are different from me now. In their busy lives they may never know as much suffering, isolation or pain as me. They may never see beyond what is well-known, conventional and safe.

Without you, M.E., I might never have been lost in the wilderness. Without you, M.E., I might never have found myself there either.

I sign off,

Elizabeth Guntrip

POTS, EDS, AND FIBROMYALGIA – ELLIE WHITING

Dear Postural Orthostatic Tachycardia, Ehlers-Danlos Syndrome and Fibromyalgia,

First off, where on Earth did you all come from?! It's as if one day I woke up without the ability to stand without passing out. My joints began to make themselves known to me, and all of a sudden I was feeling the heat of foreign countries whilst still being in dreary England.

It was so quick. I used to be able to dance and walk home from days out in town. Now I can't walk around a supermarket unaided, and for that, I hate you. I used to play Rounders at school and go to parties at the weekend, dancing and laughing until the small hours. Now I struggle to shower and can't socialise for more than an hour, and for that, I hate you. I used to spend time outside, seeing things and hanging out with friends. Now I spend most of my time in doctors' rooms, being tested in bizarre ways and told my conditions are incurable, and for that, I really hate you. Especially after getting me in the situation of eating radioactive mashed potato at 10 a.m. and drinking barium liquid which can only be described as sherbet, cement, and chalk in a cup.

Despite everything you have taken away from me, I have to give you credit for what you have shown me. I now appreciate the importance of friends and realise who is worth sticking around for, who will hold my hand and wipe my tears when it's a bad day, and who will push my wheelchair without an ounce of shame. I can now appreciate the little things. For instance, sometimes sitting on a bench by the duck pond is the highlight of my day, because I'm out of my bed and I'm well enough to hold myself in a sitting position. I have learnt to immerse myself in the moment too, taking in all the sounds, the smells, and the people I am with, and truly appreciating what I am able to experience. You have also helped me overcome my fear of needles and vomiting, by giving me no choice about the matter, and you've managed to get me anaesthesia on more than one occasion, providing the best sleep I have ever and will ever have. Floating on marshmallow clouds with time moving so s-l-o-w-l-y really does help to ease the pain of ECGs being implanted in my chest, wires fed through my groin up to my heart and endoscopes shoved down my throat.

The hardest thing you took away from me, was my pride. Being in a wheelchair is liberating and allows me some freedom, but it's not all fun really- I used to be taller than all my friends, and now I sit at bum height. It's like a sea of bottoms when we go out! Because of you, I have endured stares and hurtful comments, been questioned about my own capability and made to feel so small yet so in the way whilst facing the difficulties of being disabled in public. Using a walking stick looks easy, but when it comes down to carrying a bag, a folder and rummaging for keys at the same time, the walking stick becomes a challenge (many a time have I whacked it against my car as I'm trying to bundle myself in). If it wasn't for you, I may have been able to gracefully leave my classroom and get in the car.

Something I want to call you out on is the impact you have had on my family. And for that, I truly despise what you have put them through. My mum, who is a nurse, continues her nursing when she gets home through looking after me, meaning she doesn't get to finish her shift or take a break. The amount of times you have kept her up with me whilst she massaged my sore, tender body, grabbed ice packs and listened to me sob, is unimaginable. My younger sister has been told to come straight home after school rather than socialise, because she has to get back to assist me due to the things YOU do to me: the crazy heart rate, the heavy head, the nausea, and the weakness that leaves me unable to get downstairs for a drink, or to dry my own hair. My grandparents have paid ridiculous sums of money in an attempt to help me, covering private specialists, multiple hotel stays for early morning hospital appointments all over London, therapists, and weekly lymphatic drainage massages. They didn't work all their lives for you to just take from them so selfishly. You simply decided to make me so unwell and desperate that those things became necessary. You see, you haven't just impacted on my life greatly, you have impacted the people closest to me and caused so much distress and helplessness.

Through all the bad, the good is still there. I am still Ellie and I always will be. I'm just an altered version of Ellie. Maybe that is a good thing: you have taught me how to truly and deeply love and not to be afraid of expressing my gratitude for the people around me. You have taught me that being disabled through chronic illness is not a life sentence to unhappiness, it's just a quirk- I don't know many friends that own a floral walking stick or have been steered around shops in a wheelchair, crashed into multiple displays and cried with laughter from it. You have taught me that drinking lemonade shots whilst my friends necked down cocktails can be just as much fun, because it's about the people surrounding me and being thankful for them, and their acceptance of me as I am, with you included. You have taught me that achieving things is possible even when people don't have faith. Changing the direction of life and goals is acceptable, being adaptable is an incredible quality and without you, I wouldn't have that.

You have changed my life in unimaginable ways, both

negative and positive, that will stay with me. Although you took my teenage years away, you replaced it with a perspective and outlook on life that's hard to come by. By the way, don't worry, when the doctors do find a cure for at least one of you, I won't forget you. Despite you landing me in many a hospital bed and making my bones pop like a bowl of Rice Krispies, you have made me a better person, and for that,

I thank you.

Ellie Whiting

LYME DISEASE AND DYSAUTONOMIA – EMMA ANDERSON

You must both sit smugly whenever someone asks me the question: "Do you wish this had never happened to you?" You know very well my answer is a surprising 'no', that I don't want to erase my time with you. It took me a long time to realise my answer is 'no' to that question but the more I thought about it, the more I saw how you've changed me for the better. How can I take back everything I've learnt now? Don't get me wrong, I don't enjoy your random outbursts, constant lifestyle restrictions and shenanigans. Has anyone ever told you how antisocial you are?! Although I admit, sometimes you can be quite the comedian: when you mince my words or add in a totally inappropriate one, I can't help but laugh.

And it's true that I'm extremely glad to be getting treatment that will begin our messy separation from our seven year relationship or rather, tolerance. No, I can honestly say I am who I am today because of you.

When we first met I was nineteen. I was struggling with anxiety over food and completely stressed out by trying and failing to balance university and social life. My mindset was fixed on working: working all hours of the day to achieve the best grades in my fashion course. My aim was to be successful and take home a good salary. I wrongly measured success by money. What a fool I was. Everything else was put aside. I passed up on so many opportunities for fun and I lost time with my friends and family that I will never get back, just to attempt to create something my tutors deemed acceptable for my prestigious London University degree. This now fills me with regret. I will never get that time back, especially with those who are no longer here or no longer in my life.

You, and only you, have taught me how to have balance. How success should never be measured by money alone. How to eat again without obsessing over calories. How to laugh when I'm full of pain. How to get up every time I fall down – quite literally! You've shown me that family and friends are equally as important as working, maybe more so. I feel privileged that in my twenties I have this insight, this knowledge that some people will only ever find in old age, when it's too late. I know now that I am not defined by my career or by my status, but by the way I treat others and my outlook on life.

You've also opened new doors for me. Some of my closest friends are ones I've found since you've been a part of my life. I could never wish to undo that. And I can't see any possibility that I would have met them without you. You've also shown me who my true friends are, and while so many people are no longer part of my life, I am now left with the amazing people who do their best to adapt to you and understand you. Although, honestly, I would never wish to formally introduce you to any of my friends. I wouldn't wish the burden of carrying you upon anyone.

Of course, at times you are isolating and our first few months together were extremely intense. You were that keen on making my body your home that I thought I might die. Even my family thought I was dying. I surprised myself that I wasn't scared, I just wanted darkness and sleep. But I lived and then improved enough not to be in bed all day. I also found out how adaptive I was, even more so when dysautonomia dramatically brought POTS into my life. What an entrance you made. I will never forget the day you stole my sight for a good ten minutes, or that sensation that came with it of not knowing up from down or left from right.

For a time we all managed to compromise but over the last three years, you've got aggressive again, to the point where you're actually starting to scare me. You invite your friend depression over a few times and I have to work double hard to get him to leave. Somehow, I manage to pull through. All this has shown me just how strong and adaptable I am.

You kept your true identities well-hidden for a long time. But I found you out. You're both smarter than most doctors I've met. I was diagnosed with Post-Viral Chronic Fatigue Syndrome/ME in 2010 but after six years, I felt I knew you well enough to pursue a different diagnosis. Doctors refused to believe in you, dysautonomia, because they just didn't know about you.

For two years I pursued a POTS diagnosis. Once I had achieved that and a chance to better my dysautonomia through medication, there was no stopping me: I decided to test privately for Lyme disease. I had a hunch that's who you really were and I was right. I knew you better than most doctors. To give you a name was wonderful, to know how you work was an insight I wish was possible for all chronic illness.

This last year, things have changed for us three. I discovered the full extent of dysautonomia, for which I started oxygen therapy to reset my autonomic system. I felt a tiny bit stronger within days and even stronger now, after four months of treatment. And Lyme, I'm on month four of attacking you with antibiotics. I feel for once things are shifting and not down into the darkness anymore. Because of you two, I have to take seven lots of medications a day, which amounts to sixty pills and liquids. If you picked me up I might rattle!

You might not like my poor treatment of you now, but I'm desperate to face the real world again. I know I'll be safe with the knowledge you taught me. These life lessons I will never forget.

I know you won't leave me easily and that I might never be totally free of you, I accept that. But I really hope in time this relationship will fade, like so many do. I hope you can free me to be an even better version of what you've made me today.

Emma

LYME DISEASE – FAYE SAVORY

Dear Lyme Disease,

We've been living together for a while now. You were a quiet tenant to start with but once you'd settled in, you really made your presence known. Since I learned your name, I've tried my best to get to know you.

If I'm honest though, I don't feel like you've tried to get to know me.

In the interest of fairness, here are a few things you should know:

- I love making myself a nice cup of tea.
- I love to travel and to wander in new places.
- I love everything about festivals; the atmosphere, the music, the people.
- I love to run.
- I love being able to provide for myself financially.
- I love driving.
- I love long, hot, non-dizzy bubble baths.
- I love chocolate. I *really* love chocolate.
- I love learning a new language.
- I love being around my friends.
- I love the cinema.
- I love going out to eat.
- I love walking my dog.
- I love my home and looking after it.
- I love cooking.

- I love feeling in charge of my own life.
- I want to help people.
- I want to help people, help people.
- I want to start something.
- I want to call it BearHugs.
- I want it to be a social enterprise.
- I want to help people send packages that will brighten someone's day.
- I want to send treats to seriously ill children.
- I want to help other people with difficult tenants like you find work and ways to express themselves.
- I want to learn how to do all of this.

I don't know if it's intentional, but you seem to be making all these things as difficult as possible for me.

I'll give you a bit of time to get your things in order. But if you can't bring yourself to change then I'm afraid I might have to go to the Citizen's Advice Bureau.

Respectfully yours,

Faye Savory

BRAIN TUMOUR – GRACE LATTER

Dear...you,

Isn't that odd? I still, even when sitting alone, typing on my laptop and not actually saying anything aloud, will avoid saying that word. I can't address you properly. The correct term, the one my specialists and surgeon frequently throw around when speaking with me and other patients like me is, well, a bit hideous. Sorry, I don't mean to offend. It's just an ugly word. It looks menacing written down, and it sounds sickly when you say it out loud.

I think it's the wet 'chooo' sound it begins with, and the lazy 'murrrhhh' that ends it. It's funny, literally, because 'humour' is not dissimilarly spelled and yet has a much cleaner sound and lovelier meaning. Same with 'tuna', although I've never eaten it so I can't say if that name is appropriately nice.

Most days, I'll refer to you as 'The Thing'. If I'm feeling brave? 'That Thing in my head'. Once, when I was among friends – and a little tipsy, therefore more confident – I called you 'my pesky growth'.

I loathe the effect the hated word has on others. I'll tell someone who doesn't know already, and force myself to spit out the T-word, and the reactions are varied but generally *big*. Whether it's a gasp of horror, a heavy understanding nod, a desperate clamour for more information straight away, or an uncomfortable shift of gaze. I often find myself raising my hands up, palms out, and reassuring the person I'm telling that 'It's not that bad,' or 'I'm fine though, I'm fine!'

We give the word so much power, and with all the bad press it gets, it's no wonder. 'Fear of a name only increases fear of the thing itself'. I think the reason I avoid it like the plague – another thing which you kind of are, sorry – is because it sounds so *serious*. It can't be said gently. I've tried saying it with a light tone, just throwing it casually into a conversation – that didn't work. I've tried muttering it and hoping it just blends into the general noise of a sentence...nope. I type it and it glares at me from the page as I continue writing.

The thing is, Thing, I have to live with you for the rest of my life. I should really get used to calling you by your correct name. Well, if I'm being pedantic, I could say your scientifically accurate name, which is Grade 1 Pilocytic Astrocytoma... wow, even *that* is better than using the generic term you and your more dangerous friends all reside under. It sounds almost sparkly in comparison. Maybe because an Astrocytoma is literally star-like, in that it's a somewhat spread-out...*Thing*...that spans many layers of the brain, rather than just sitting stoutly in one spot as others tend to.

Anyway, yes, I am stuck with you. You're stuck *in* me. Although a fair bit of you has been carefully extracted and severed off and drained and bottled – there's still an indisputable part of you left to fester, and hopefully not thrive. You're still in there. You're still attached to me, in perhaps my most brilliant and dangerous and personal and fragile area. I've accepted that, as have my family and friends. I'll never be without you. So, really, yes, I should get used to saying your name and I should be comfortable uttering that ugly word. Hopefully, someday I will be.

Until then, you're my Thing. Whether I like it or not.

I'll see you soon, I'm sure – on a monitor in the oncologist's consult room. So keep behaving, please. You're doing well these days, and looking good. Don't ruin that.

Grace. X

M.E AND EHLERS-DANLOS SYNDROME – KATE STANFORTH

Dear ME and EDS,

I didn't think that twenty-two-year-old me would ever need full-time care, or that it would have been that way for nearly a decade now, but here we are. But, I wanted to thank you. Thank you for the incredible laughs I've had tackling these illnesses. Thank you for the opportunities I would never have had. Thank you, because by battling you ever so hard every day, you have made me into the strong person I am today.

I'm awoken by my care agency carer every morning, usually as she hops onto my bed and says 'Rise and shine, sunshine!' Usually, this is when I do my little growl and pull the covers over my face, grumpy at the fact I have to fight through another day. I look up, and there is my porridge. Today, the fruit has been cut out so it's in the shape of a dog. You see, my dad and my carers have a competition to see who can come up with the best porridge designs (I've even made a collage!) so I always am surprised by my work of art in the morning. I down my half a litre of water so that I don't faint when I wake up, throw back the tablets like they're smarties, and get ready for the day.

Being chronically ill means that your second home is the hospital. I really wish they did a loyalty card scheme or something, because gosh, I'm there a lot. So, today's trip is (surprise, surprise) another hospital appointment, approximately number 204,759,372. The journey there is always made hysterical by my carer though. I get anxious about these things. Despite going to hospital nearly every day, I still worry, but she sure takes my mind off it. Today, we had Adele karaoke on the way there. Love it!

We get to the hospital and it's physiotherapy time. My carer 'spectates' whilst I work my bum off for the next hour. My version of 'working my bum off' is probably a little different to yours, mind. My body struggles just with standing up so we do a lot of floor work. My favourite kind of work. We laugh at all the daft things I've done this week, like how my ankle is swollen because I ran my electric wheelchair into a lamppost at 6 mph (I was racing my two-year-old nephew by the way - I won, for the record). I also got the chair stuck down a kerb, so had to get my dad to rescue me… apparently, I'm a total liability.

On the way home I'm exhausted, and usually flat both physically and emotionally. That's when my carer and I usually talk a load of rubbish and we end up laughing all the way home.

It's lunchtime now, so she tucks me up on my recliner with the curtains shut, heated blanket on, legs elevated, tea next to me and my hot meal. I nibble at that for a while and then I'm left to nap for a few hours - phew.

The evening starts and my amazing family come home. My dad comes into my room and genuinely acts out his day in song and dance. He's not a dancer or a singer. I have no idea why he does this but it does make me smile. We email each other silly jokes through the day. I'm currently trying to convince him to get a pet rabbit so I keep sending him pictures of them to his work email and he has to open them. He's put my email into his junk box now, but that's another story. Anyways, my mum comes in and I always get so much love from her. We usually laugh about how dramatic my day has been (and I'm not going to lie, I'm usually in hysterical tears) but we comfort each other. I hear a massive knock at the door...

"IT'S ME! I'M HERE."

My two-year-old nephew makes *the* most dramatic entrances known to mankind. If he doesn't act when he grows up, I will be very shocked. He waddles in and gives me a huge cuddle.

'Auntie Kate is poorly so we have to give her lots of hugs and kisses,' he says to his mum (my sister) every day. It's hard to explain to a two-year-old that you're the type of poorly that doesn't get better, but he's so good at understanding. My sister usually takes him downstairs after a few minutes as he's a bit loud for me, and I have a rest. So there's my family care team, all arriving at once!

My boyfriend comes over later on. I'm forever laughing with him. I can't imagine how hard it is to love someone who you can see is in visible discomfort every day and you can't do anything about it, but he and my family do as much as they can to make me as happy and as comfortable as possible. I usually spend my evenings giving back. I absolutely love volunteering and I spend a lot of my time trying to help others in whatever way I can. I set up Project Parent, which gives gift boxes to the parents of poorly children in hospital over Christmas, which takes up a lot of my time. I absolutely love it and have an amazing team. I have won my first award and got two grants from O2 Think Big, which is one of my greatest achievements to date. Before this, I was a mentor for Vinspired, which was also one of the most incredible opportunities. I volunteer for lots of causes, particularly locally, from fundraising to campaigning. I've had so many opportunities with it - from travelling, to doing crazy things like zip wiring off the Tyne Bridge and indoor skydiving! But not all of these things are organised events. Last night I was making a Valentine's card and ended up making ten extra ones with gifts. These were for those who had recently become single or were having a particularly hard time at the moment. If I hadn't become ill, I wouldn't have started making jewellery and crafts when I was bedbound, which eventually led me to do an A-level in textiles and get the highest mark in the college with an A*. I'm so passionate about crafting now! And, I love doing Random Acts of Kindness. If I put a smile on anyone's face, then that makes me happy! I always wonder if I would have volunteered if I hadn't become ill, but I certainly wouldn't have done most of these things!

I have lost an awful lot through illness, from independence to friends. But I'm filling those gaps with other things and I think that's the way to tackle it. I've got a handful of amazing close friends, many of which live many miles away, but it was worth waiting this long to find these gems. I'm starting to gain a little bit of independence using my new electric chair but everything else I just try to fill with things and people I love. It's hard being ill. I paint one very brave face for most people, especially on social media where people do see me as the 'happy, positive Kate' who can take on the world, but I do cry every day. But do you know what? That's okay. It's okay if that's how you deal with things, as long as you keep going.

ME and EDS, boy are you challenging, but thank you for opening these avenues I never would have explored. Thank you for helping me support others in similar situations fight battles I would have known nothing about. So for now, I'm just going to do what I always do. Keep my chin up, my smile on, and keep fighting.

Kate x

M.E – KRISTINA LEWIS

Dear M.E,

First and foremost, I'd like to thank you. Yes, you read that right, I'm *thanking* you.

I know that might seem bizarre, given the circumstances, but a thank you is exactly what you deserve.

I'd like to thank you for showing me how strong I can be.

If I could turn the clock back eighteen years, you'd see a small brown-haired, blue-eyed girl with a beaming smile and huge dreams. A love of singing, dancing and acting that grew with every class, every audition and every opportunity. A continued determination that culminated in being awarded a scholarship to train professionally full-time in Musical Theatre. But you had other plans.

It was difficult to accept my body and mind didn't quite see eye-to-eye, but this brown-haired and blue-eyed girl is still smiling, despite the setbacks.

I'd like to thank you for showing me who my real friends are over the last few years. You've reminded me just who isn't worth my energy (what little of it I have…) or time.

You've even provided me with a group of friends who understand how it feels to be beyond exhausted every day and have also heard the same old sayings over again, from "Chronic Fatigue? Yeah, I've got that too!" to "Why don't you try *insert name of miracle cure here*?"

These girls are the friendliest and most compassionate people and I've never even met them in person!

Thank you for highlighting how even more crazy my family are!

My mum has always encouraged and supported me with everything, and we've got so many hilarious memories together, whilst my sister, Charlene, and brother, Barry, along with my nieces and nephews, Jack, Phoebe, Ben and Chloe, never fail to make me laugh or put a smile on my face. My boyfriend, Tom, also goes above and beyond to help me on a daily basis, from cooking my meals to being my personal chauffeur service when I'm not well enough to drive myself. I even get treated to sing-a-long sessions to cheer me up – although he's not quite mastered some of the Musical soundtracks yet. Sorry, Tom! ;)

M.E, I certainly can't forget to thank you for all the new opportunities you've provided me with.

A few years ago, my Mum reminded me of a project I had worked on as a child, a voiceover for a series for Fox Kids TV. I loved being in the voiceover booth, bringing my character to life with an infectious giggle. That Christmas, my Mum surprised me with a place on a voiceover training course. She provided me with the greatest opportunity to perform again, albeit in an alternative way.

Since then, I've been able to voice animations, apps and audiobooks from home, including for well-known companies such as The National Trust, Benefit Cosmetics UK, and the World Health Organisation. Voice acting allows me the opportunity to perform, something which I will never stop.

You enabled me to volunteer for a number of projects, including Project Parent, a non-profit initiative set up by my now good friend and fellow M.E sufferer, Kate. Project Parent provides gift boxes to parents with children in hospital at Christmas in Newcastle, Bristol, Lancaster, Leeds, and Southampton. I have been lucky enough to become the leader for the Bristol area and have worked with my fellow leaders, volunteers and fundraisers to deliver boxes for two years running. This has been such an eye-opening experience and it just wouldn't have happened without you! I certainly can't wait for my third Christmas with the team!

I've been lucky enough to be selected to represent Team Wales in the first ever Paracheer Freestyle Pom division at the International Cheerleading Union World Championships in Florida, this April. Paracheer divisions comprise of teams with a mixture of disabled and able-bodied athletes.

I've worked hard to build up my strength to enable me to compete with this team and I'm so excited to represent my country on their Worlds Stage.

Obviously, thanks to you, I still have particularly bad days (sometimes too frequently for my liking!), but after you've been around so long, I've learnt to deal with you in the best ways I can.

Competing in this way certainly doesn't mean that I'm not still ill; it's a demonstration of my determinism and how hard I've worked to be able to achieve these opportunities.

These thank-you's will only continue to grow whilst you're accompanying me on my journey and I can't wait to see what you inspire me to do next.

Kristina x

M.E AND POTS – LARA STRONG

Dear M.E. and POTS,

We first met when I was fourteen, when my life was all about who was dating who that week, playing netball, trying to do just enough work to get me by at school, and many, many sleepless sleepovers. I led a very lucky life. Unbeknownst to me, you had other ideas, so you kept creeping in and over those next few years, life started to look a little less careless and a lot more care home. My wonder turned from who I might be when I grow up and what I might do, to will I make it through today or the next hour, because the symptoms of you were so unbelievably bad. I went from teenager to doddery grandma in a weird Benjamin Button-esque way; feeling physically ancient despite my biological age of nineteen.

It was absolute hell, I won't lie about that. And now, at twenty-five, well, it still can be, but it's a tad easier to mentally cope with thanks to some perspective, a lot more patience and hopefully a little bit of wisdom on my side (Which I'm sure anyone in a long-term relationship such as ours could do with). That's not the only thing that's changed. Two years ago, I graduated with a law degree in my hand, one which I earnt largely from my bed (unfortunately this was thanks to you, as opposed to gross amounts of vodka). I am wildly proud of myself for this, and will always have it as a reminder of what my ill-self is still capable of. But as I look around, it hits me: people my age are moving on. They've done the uni thing and now it's onwards and upwards for them: living on their own, getting their dream job, engagements, marriage, babies even. And I'm lying here, still unable to take the first step: a job, a career.

The crazy thing is I never knew something like you even existed because no one seems to talk about the possibility of *this*. Yes, people got cancer and had heart attacks. I knew that awful stuff happened; Life and death type stuff. But not you, not the in-between life and death stuff. Young people like me getting this sick and staying there for potentially the rest of their lives, in a boring torturous limbo, which then makes it really hard for anyone to understand the phrase, "I'm twenty-five and haven't washed my hair in two weeks because I have an unpronounceable chronic illness." They can't quite believe it unless it's actually happened to them.

For a long time, an awfully long time, I kept hoping (and if I'm honest, still occasionally do) that one day I would wake up and you would be gone; realizing the suffering you had caused myself and my family, you would have realised your selfish ways and left. So when people asked what I'd been up to, I wouldn't have to tell them "Well, resting..." finished off with a few inaudible mumbles. There would be no more morning paralysis; no more aggressive vertigo which made me feel like a much less cheery Lionel Richie - talk about dancing on the ceiling; no more nagging nausea; no more nerve pain screeching down my spine; no more muscles burning because I rested my arm on a ledge (seriously, that is ridiculous, it's resting there, for goodness sake!); no more feeling as if someone had electrocuted my brain and beaten the bleep out of me in my sleep. Just normal. Not 'crazy, healthy, jumping out of bed and running a half marathon – just normal. I know, wishful thinking: gotta stay positive, right?

But hey, I know you're not a person (albeit this letter's tone is rather misleading); you're just some piece of rubbish genetic code or misbehaving mitochondria, you can't have it in for me. This is no personal vendetta, because you don't have a brain (burn!). You are, as much as I wish you weren't, just a part of me. A part of my body, which means it needs extra TLC and caution, and sometimes near-total lack of living to stay alive. You are here to stay for who-knows how long and who-knows how severely. So we've gotta ride this rollercoaster called life as best we can, together.

In our years of co-existence, you have undoubtedly taught me to live in the moment, in a world where we are obsessed with "What's next?" Little "normal" moments are like treasure to me, which I'm sure would have been invisible to a "healthy" Lara. And I love harder because of you, including myself. In fact, I love myself fiercely because I know how important it is to do so, to look after myself mentally, and to no longer correlate self-worth with the number in my bank account, or little letters next to my name. We are all just us. When you strip it back, we are all just unique souls. And that is worth something, in itself.

My new mindset is to live the life I have, to the fullest. If today I am too ill to shuffle in my usual, hunched over, "granny before her time" way to the toilet, and crawling/dragging myself is the only way, then heck, the bathroom is my Everest and I will treat it like an epic quest and awesome achievement when I reach the summit. Or If I'm lucky and I can get out for an hour or two, once a fortnight, I will laugh with my friend as much as possible and give them a giant squeeze hello. And I will always be indescribably grateful for the love and care of my family, my foundation, whom I fear I might have overlooked in an alternate healthy universe.

Now don't get it twisted, M.E., there are still many days, as I'm sure you've noticed, when I will mentally mutter 'eff-this' a thousand times. I will think 'I just can't do this anymore, what's the point?' And then I'll bring myself back from the edge, as always. Like a Mum talking to her kid, I'll tell myself and my poor battered body, 'It's going to be okay, this isn't it. There's so much life still to be lived, so many smiles and laughs to be heard and had. So don't you dare give up, got it?'

So, my old frenemy M.E., you really have been quite the gloomy old cloud over my life but like the clichéd saying, you have your silver linings and what I've come to realize is that I still lead a very lucky life in every possible way, despite you.

Yours unfortunately but acceptingly,

Lara

SEVERE M.E – MERETE GRAHAM

Dear Severe Myalgic Encephalomyelitis.

Thank you for dragging me through the hardest times of my life. Without you, I would never have stumbled upon my inner strength, my power and my inner spark.

You see, while you were tearing my body down, steady and targeted, I was learning things life could not in any other way have taught me.

First of all, I learned how severe M.E. is very different from "just being a little tired". Even after living with M.E. for years, I couldn't in my wildest imagination understand the scope of this particular illness. In a very short time and quite brutally, if I may say so myself, I learned how severe M.E. could take away my life in so many aspects. Being bedridden and relying on help for everything from getting dressed and eating, to personal hygiene and going to the toilet in a wheelchair, is unbearable for a girl in her early twenties. I've been bedridden for three years, which means I've also been unable to see my friends and family. Truth be told, I feel like I've lost almost every one of all the beautiful people I had in my life, during this time.

This is heart-breaking and almost impossible to wrap your head around, isn't it? But on top of all of this, you were going to make me stare death in the eye. I never expected you to be so cruel, dear M.E. Actually, I'm still staring death in the eye every single day. My life-line is the tube that comes out of my chest. Hooked up to my heart, I now get nutrition directly into the blood as you, dear ME, have made my body completely unable to tolerate any food. You even tricked all the doctors to believe I had tons of other illnesses, but all the time it was you. A devious one you are indeed. But I thank you, dear ME, because you've taught me things beyond my imagination and way beyond my age.

You've taught me deep compassion, honesty and love. You've taught me to see life from a new perspective and you've taught me to never judge anyone I meet because I know nothing about the fights they are facing in their lives.

You've taught me to see actions instead of words, connection instead of difference, and souls instead of titles or names.

You've taught me that seeing your life crumble apart between your hands is an opportunity to find your inner light and follow it. To rise up.

You have taught me that losing five, ten or even twenty friends can break your world, but in the end, it means nothing as long as you have that one special friend that will never let you down. You've taught me to open up, speak up and lead. You've taught me to become a new person, a better version of myself. And for that, I thank you.

I would never ever wish this illness upon anyone, not even my worst enemy, and my biggest hope and wish is to wake up healthy. Every single day when I wake up, before I open my eyes, I hope this is the day I'm stepping out of my living hell, and back into my life. I'm still waiting for that day to come, but I will never lose hope.

Also, the strength I've gained, the lessons you've taught me, dear ME, is something I would never exchange for anything else. All the beautiful friends this illness has brought into my life from within the spoonie community; I didn't know you guys existed. I wouldn't have been here today without your love and support through all of this, especially through those life-threatening times where I was overwhelmed with fear and needed love more than anything.

So, dear ME, thank you for making my life a living hell, so I could light my inner spark. Thank you for teaching me how to create my own rays of lights in the midst of darkness.

Kindest regards,
Merete Graham

M.E – NIKKI GITTINS

Dear M.E.

You may be a pain in my bum but we have been through a lot together over the years and I have come to accept you for who you are. Who else would I have to thank for my appreciation of snuggle wear (pyjamas to 'normal' people), love of blankets, and the weird secret snacking that occurs when the sleeping tablets have kicked in a bit, but not enough to send me to sleep - many a fond memory we have shared. We may have had our rocky roads, from the first time we visited the hospital together all those years ago to having you repeatedly question my ability to continue education - I believe it is three nil to me, but who's counting?

We met seventeen years ago. It was summer and I was busy with exams, but within a week of meeting you, you were soon taking up all of my time. We would spend the days sleeping and the nights snuggled up in bed, watching films. You and I would travel to all the different doctors, health professionals and hospitals in the local area. After six months and countless opinions, no one could figure out our relationship. Were we just unlucky or was there a reason for our connection? Nobody could seem to figure it out.

After months, we chanced upon someone who we would later find to be our saviour, our counsellor to navigate the stormy seas of our difficult marriage. She would see both of our points of view, even when my eyes were closed. Back then, I didn't want to know, so I just pushed against you like a child against a well-meaning parent. It would be years before I began to appreciate that you were trying to protect me with your warning signs and mold me into the person I have become.

Over the years we have had our laughs, including the time my tutors had bad news for me but you had me so drugged up I couldn't have cared less, leaving them not knowing what to think. And then there are our nocturnal taxi trips to surgeries and A&E. I think my friend, who joined us on one of our adventures, particularly enjoyed celebrating her birthday in Accident and Emergency.

As the years have passed, society has become more accepting and accommodating of our relationship, trying to help us manage daily tasks easier; some people may call it a Blue Badge, but to us, it is VIP parking (and a lifeline). People who don't know us sometimes question the validity of our relationship, but the people who truly know us see our connection every day. They help us enjoy and celebrate our good days and they support us through the tough ones. And let's be honest, there have been some tough ones. Luckily we have learned a mutual language in which to communicate; we know the difference between 'tired', 'shattered' and 'exhausted'. To some, they may be similar, but to us the differences are vast. Tired means we need to have a nap during the day, shattered is us not being able to concentrate on anything properly and needing to go to bed, and exhausted... well, all bets are off and we struggle to get out of the cosy nest we call the snuggle fortress. These are the days where I truly appreciate the fragility of our mutual understanding, always teetering, wobbling like a child's play toy.

You have brought out the quirks in me, some of which I never knew I had... The need to immediately change into pyjamas as soon as we get through the front door; my ability to binge-watch a TV series, yet films seem like too much 'work'; and my affinity with 'old lady' culture: extra layers, comfy clothes, early bedtimes and great appreciation of hot beverages. You have taught me to embrace the inner weirdo, whose love for unicorns, rainbows and super cute things is only recently being copied by fashionistas. Thanks to you I have learnt to become confident in my own skin and identity, remembering that being different is interesting and a lot of fun.

A relationship like ours could make some people very sad and back in the early days, I struggled mentally and emotionally with our connection. I did not like that you were constantly there, overbearing me, so controlling in your ways. As time has moved on though and we have both grown, you have taught me to look on the bright side of life, laugh at myself and be happy with what I have. That is not to say we don't still have rough patches, but we work through them, knowing that we are bound together, and one of us will probably pay the other back if we carry on fighting...

Over the years we have been through five homes, three degrees, one relationship, several friends, countless doctors and enough medication to stock a pharmacy. There are many times when I wish I had never met you, but then there are the times when I appreciate what you have brought into my life; the support network, the wonderful spoonie community, the determination, the lateral career path, the ability to help others and above all, the assurance in myself.

So thank you, Myalgic Encephalomyelitis, for allowing me to prove you wrong on so many occasions and teaching me what it is like to be human but, as I said at the start, you are a pain in my bum.

Nikki

M.E AND POTS – OLIVIA COLE

Dear M.E and POTS

Just thought I'd write to you and tell you that it's been eight years now, though I'm sure you're both very aware of this, as you live with me every single day and have changed my life both for the worse and better.

For the past eight years you've put me in situations I didn't think would be possible or fair for a little unwell girl to go through. You've shown me the true meaning behind the word disbelief by putting me right in front of the people that show it and let me tell you now, that isn't a fun experience for a ten-year-old girl. But now I am an eighteen-year-old woman and you have shown me how to appreciate the small but near insignificant things in life and for this, I am forever grateful.

Never could I of imagined that my childhood and teenage years would have been snatched away from me so suddenly and for this, I shall never forgive you. But you see, you've taught me that sometimes life doesn't go as expected. It's what you make of it and how you choose to get through it that is most important. As long as you appreciate the trees and the people that stick by you every day, you really will be okay.

Although I feel like I could now make a great sequel to the Groundhog Day movie, I'm hoping that the rest of my life won't be that way. Because of you, I had the idea to set up a page to unite people from all around the world that are in the same situation. As a result, I am now lucky enough to have spoken to hundreds of others like me.

The page is called CFS Selfies and it has made my ongoing experience so much easier. I didn't quite realise how much it would when I initially set it up. I was just hoping for a few people to send me a photo of themselves on a good (well, enough to get out of bed) day and then on a bad day (days where we are bedridden and can't do anything). I hoped that it would help bring us together, so that we would be able to compare symptoms and try to make light of this situation that we have found ourselves in. But I have met some amazing people and have been shown the true strength, courage and positivity of M.E sufferers. This has been truly incredible and makes me so happy!

I also got the chance to appear on Good Morning Britain to help raise awareness of you, M.E, as healthy people still do not realise how life-crushing you truly are. However, by us sufferers and our families speaking out, we are gradually getting there, baby-step by baby-step. Crazy what a good and bad day photo can do, hey?!

Chronic illness, you really are a pain both literally and physically, but I'm excited to see where life takes me as a wiser person. Living with you is like living every day with an extremely, unreasonably controlling person. One day though, you won't control me.

Best wishes

Olivia Cole

EDS, FIBROMYALGIA, AND POTS – SARAH ALEXANDER

Dear Ehlers-Danlos Syndrome, Fibromyalgia and Postural Tachycardia Syndrome,

Wow, could you have at least been shorter words or easier to pronounce? Could you not have made that easy on me? If I had a pound for every time I had to spell you, I can guarantee I'd be a very rich woman.

I used to hate you, I used to wish you weren't part of my life; I used to want to be 'normal'. But what's 'normal'? My normal includes pain. Every single day I'm in pain. Some days it's worse than others but it's always there, it's always in the background, waiting to jump up and take over. Waiting for me to stretch a little bit further or do a tiny bit more than usual, and there it is, climbing on my back, pulling a joint out of its socket, tearing a ligament, damaging a tendon, controlling my every move.

Even when I'm having a low pain day, you're on my mind; I can't get away from you. And EDS, I'm looking at you, since you affect my collagen; you play havoc with my bowel, bladder, heart and head; as well as my muscles, joints, ligaments, tendons, skin and blood. Can I catch a break? Actually no, don't throw 'a break' at me. Knowing my luck, I'll end up even more broken.

It's really tough; I spend a lot of time with tears running down my cheeks because the pain is taking over my everything. You'd think I'd be used to it after almost twenty years, and in a way I am. I know it'll always be there, I'm well aware that my conditions won't miraculously disappear, but I also never expected it to be as bad as it is. A part of me forgets the torture of a flare-up: the frustration, the anger, the sadness. A flare is like an abyss, as there's no end in sight at the beginning, it completely consumes me and there are times I've wished for death. But there's always a flicker of hope. It could be something my boyfriend says, a picture of my nephew that turns my frown into a smile, a day of slightly less pain, a good night's sleep, anything. And it helps me to remember all the times I've got through this before. Every single time I've been here, I've fought my way out of it. Sometimes I've just ridden it out, but I've come out the other end.

I've not even mentioned the fatigue. Do you know how exhausting it is to be in pain 24/7, too much pain even to sleep? It's such a vicious cycle. I used to feel guilty for sleeping late but now I don't care, I just go to bed late and wake up whenever I want. I feel like I'll be tired for the rest of my life but luckily I have some excellent beauty products to help conceal the eye-bags.

For me, the worst part about having a chronic illness is feeling like a burden. I require a lot of help in every aspect of my life. My boyfriend helps me wash and get dressed. He cooks, cleans and generally does most things, and I sometimes feel like his life revolves around me so much that it'd be easier for him if we had never met. I've obviously spoken to him about it and he completely disagrees because I'm a constant delight (sense the sarcasm?) to be around. However, it's really difficult when you see other couples doing things you'd never be able to do. I guess it helps that I'm great company and absolutely hilarious though, or why else would he wash my hair?

Another thing I don't like about you is the uncertainty. I can never say 'yes' for definite to a plan. I constantly rearrange or have to go home early. I've lost touch with so many people because of you and it's really tough. I know if they didn't stick around they probably weren't worth it but being reliable is a quality a lot of people look for in a pal and I'm not that because of my illnesses. I'm getting this pacing thing under my belt though, and I plan my weeks with military precision and that seems to help. I now know to never shower and wash my hair on days that I'm actually doing something because it not only exhausts me but it bloody kills. Instead, I'll do it the day before so I can rest for the remainder of the day, and have a longer, better time out when I do go. Its small adjustments that I've noticed have made massive differences, and I plan on continuing to learn what works for me.

If only I could learn how to prevent flares for the rest of my life...but I guess that's way too much of a big ask.

I don't want to be in pain every day. I don't want to spend my days cooped up in my house unable to participate in society. I don't want to visit hospitals more than my loved ones. But do you know what? I've accepted it and I've chosen not to dwell on it. Yes, I dislocate daily, I fall over a lot, I can't put my own socks on and I can't think straight half of the time, but I also wouldn't be who I am without my chronic illnesses. I wouldn't have had any of the opportunities I've had without my disability. I wouldn't know all of the beautiful people I do.

My chronic conditions have made me into a strong, determined woman who is extremely passionate about disability rights and raising awareness. They've taught me compassion, empathy and the value of true friendship; and even though they hurt like hell, mess with my heart, and feel like I've been hit in the head with a brick, I wouldn't be me without them.

I don't hate you, EDS, Fibro and POTS, but I don't think we'll ever be best friends.

Yours forever,

Sarah Alexander

THE END

FURTHER INFORMATION

Thanks for reading! Keep up with me and my latest work at www.lifeofpippa.co.uk, or say hello on Twitter: I'm at @lifeofpippa_.

To find out more about the organisations mentioned in this book, please visit the following:

Spoonie Survival Kits: www.spooniesurvivalkits.com

Project Parent: www.projectparentgb.com

BearHugs Gifts: bearhugsgifts.com

CFS Selfies: http://www.cfsselfies.com/

If you would like support for any of the conditions mentioned in this book, the following charities may be able to help:

ME/CFS: www.actionforme.org.uk

Fibromyalgia: www.fmauk.org

POTS: www.potsuk.org

Lyme Disease: www.lymediseaseaction.org.uk

Brain Tumour: www.thebraintumourcharity.org

Endometriosis: www.endometriosis-uk.org

Ehlers-Danlos Syndrome: www.ehlers-danlos.org

Dysautonomia: www.dysautonomiainternational.org

If you have concerns about your condition or general health, always talk to a medical professional involved in your care.

Chronic illness can be an isolating experience for many. If you are struggling with mental illness or thoughts of suicide, please talk to somebody. The Samaritans are a wonderful support system available 24/7, and can be contacted by calling 116 123 (UK) or emailing jo@samaritans.org. There are further accessibility options for the helpline on The Samaritans website, at www.samaritans.org. Please know that you matter, and that you are never alone.

If you struggle to get out but would like to connect with other chronically ill young people, using the internet can be a wonderful way to do so: Scope's Online Community is a thriving digital forum for talking about all things disability, and can be found at community.scope.org.uk. Social media is also an amazing way to meet new people: check out hashtags such as #spoonie, #chronicillness and #disability to find others on Facebook, Twitter and Instagram, and get involved with the chronic illness community. We're a friendly bunch!

Printed in Great Britain
by Amazon